Wheat Belly Diet: Fact Or Fiction

Lose Fat, Get Lean in Less Time!

By Patricia Steele

Exclusive Bonus Resource for Readers of the Wheat Belly Diet: Fact Or Fiction

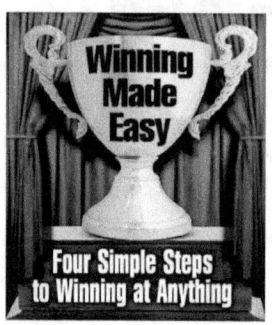

✔ Discover the 4 Steps to Winning Everyday in Every Way in your life!

✔ Learn how you can make money consistently and effortlessly.

✔ Get insider secrets to attracting and keeping your soul mate happy!

Table of Contents

Contents

Table of Contents...2
Introduction...4
A Few Statistics on Obesity..4
   Who Cares About Statistics? 4
An Introduction to the Wheat Belly Diet...6
   Rise of WHEAT Consumption in the Modern Diet...6
   Understanding Wheat...8
The Wheat Belly Diet: What Is It? 10
   Get Ready for Better Health 10
   Wheat Elimination Is Only the First Step..11
   Going Cold Turkey 12
   Plan for Success 12
   The Side Effects of Reintroducing Wheat 13
   Taking Your Weight Loss to the Next Level..13
   What to Eat 15
Is This Diet Right For Me? 17
Wheat Belly vs Healthy Eating and Exercise 18
Tips to Succeed with the WHEAT Belly Diet 19
Conclusion 20

Introduction

The weight loss industry has become one of the biggest industries in the world, with billions of dollars being spent every year. In fact, Market Data Enterprises, a market research firm specializing in the U.S. weight loss market that has spent the past 33 years tracking this market, has revealed that they expect the weight loss market to be worth $66 billion in 2013, which translates into a growth of 4.5 percent.

And that's just the U.S.!

The weight loss industry was one of the few industries that did not experience a contraction during the recession. It didn't grow but it didn't fall either. However, increased stress levels and a lower amount of available income to spend on healthy foods and weight loss programs has led to an increase in the number of overweight and obese people. In other words, people are getting fatter and are more desperate than ever to find a way to shed the pounds.

A Few Statistics on Obesity

Obesity has become a serious problem in modern society. In fact, it's now being referred to as an epidemic and it's easy to understand why. According to the World Health Organization, the cases of obesity have doubled on a global scale since 1980. In 2008, more than 1.4 billion people older than 20 were overweight, with more than a third being considered obese. In other words, 35 percent of adults were overweight and 11 percent were obese. And things have only gotten worse since 2008.

The same report shows that there were more than 40 million overweight children under the age of five in 2011. Another interesting fact is that 65 percent of people live in countries where more people die from being overweight and obese than they do from starvation. According to the WHO, at least 2.8 million adults die every year from being overweight or obese. Additionally, 44 percent of diabetes cases, 23 percent of ischemic heart disease cases and between 7 and 41 percent of certain cancer cases are caused by excess weight.

Being overweight or obese, as defined by the WHO, is having abnormal or excessive levels of fat accumulation that could cause health problems. According to the same organization, anyone with a BMI equal to or higher than 25 is overweight, while a BMI of 30 or higher signifies obesity.

Who Cares About Statistics?

You might be wondering what obesity statistics and the size of the weight loss industry have to do with losing weight. Why talk about these numbers when we should be looking at the Wheat Belly Diet, right? Well, these numbers help put things into perspective.

The size of the weight loss industry says one thing: people are lazy. It's true. We all want instant gratification. Don't shake your head because you know it's true. We all know exactly what it takes to lose weight but we don't like it. We just hate the idea of going to the gym and getting all hot and sweaty or puffing like a steam train during a workout. We hate the idea of eating nothing but lettuce leaves and celery sticks.

Instead, we want an easy way to shed those pounds quickly and painlessly, which is why everyone keeps on searching for the magic pill to drop the pounds overnight, if possible.

The amount of money being spent on weight loss programs, pills, diet books, gadgets and gizmos is obscene. Think about how many people could be fed with the amount of money we spend on looking for magic solutions to lose weight.

In other words, we're spending a fortune on things that, essentially, tell us to eat less while there are people out there who are starving.

This is probably not what you expected to read in a diet book but this should help you gain a little perspective on what the weight loss industry is really based on. There is no such thing as a magic solution to weight loss because if there were, we'd all look like Victoria's Secret models or fitness models for the guys, and $66 billion wouldn't be spent every year on new products to help us lose weight and keep it off.

That doesn't mean some of the stuff being sold doesn't work. It just means that we have issues because we buy diet books, diet pills, weight loss shakes, exercise equipment, gym memberships and the latest gizmo that will track everything from how many calories we burn to how many times we pee, yet we never, ever follow through.

And companies know that. That's why they are popping out product after product knowing that we'll all rush out to buy the next shiny thing that comes along, hoping that we can shed fifty pounds in three days, preferably without moving our rear ends off the couch. If we can eat chocolate as well, then that's the perfect diet. Right?

So, in this book we will definitely analyze the Wheat Belly Diet and see whether it's worth doing or not. However, the fact is that if you don't follow through and actually **take action**, then you are never going to lose weight, no matter how many books, pills or gizmos you buy.

A Primer on the Wheat Belly Diet

The Wheat Belly Diet was created by Dr. William Davis and made popular by the book of the same name. Dr. Davis essentially demonizes wheat, claiming that it's the main culprit behind the large numbers of obese people in the world. And he has provided some evidence to back up his statements.

So, let's take a look at why wheat might actually be bad for you and why it might be the main cause for your excess weight.

Rise of WHEAT Consumption in the Modern Diet

Wheat has always been a significant part of the human diet. In fact, the consumption of this grain in various forms is an ingrained ritual and it's so prevalent that it's even worked its way into the language. For example, if something is as good as "sliced bread", it's considered to be amazing. If you "take the bread from someone's mouth", you are taking away something that's absolutely necessary to them. If you are "the bread winner of the family, you are bringing in the family income. If you are considered "the upper crust", you are maybe a part of high society. There are plenty more examples besides these.

Wheat even features in many religious rituals, showing exactly how important bread and wheat are to human culture all over the world. There isn't a country that doesn't have some form of bread that is an important dietary staple, from the Italian ciabatta and the Greek pita, to the Indian flatbread and the sliced white bread in the United States.

So, this makes it difficult to believe that something that is so essential to many of us could actually bad for us. The problem is that today's wheat and bread have little to do with what our ancestors used to eat. Wheat has changed significantly from the original strains of wild grass humans used to harvest. Now there are more than 25,000 varieties of wheat, thanks to human tinkering.

While the beginning of the 20th century saw major changes to the grinding of wheat as it became more mechanized, the grain itself remained the same. This all changed towards the end of the 20th century, when an increase in hybridization methods changed wheat completely. In fact, a close analysis of some of the strains of wheat that are grown today will show they have little in common with the original grain.

The goal of this genetic tinkering was to create wheat that delivered a higher yield, cost less to produce and offered a consistent harvest. Essentially, the idea is for companies to make a higher profit with no one stopping to question whether or not these changes would have an impact on human health.

So, while a loaf of bread made from today's wheat might look the same and even taste similar to what our grandmothers used to bake, on a biochemical level they are completely different.

A small change to the protein structure of this grain can lead to a terrible immune response in the human body, even if our system had no immune response to the original grain.

In other words, the human body had no problems whatsoever in digesting grain for thousands of years but once we started tinkering with it and changing its molecular structure, many of us experience an allergic reaction to it, even if we don't realize it.

What Dr. Davis emphasizes is that real wheat isn't bad for us. It's the grain that has been genetically modified by agricultural companies to generate higher profits that's harmful, especially considering that it has little in common with what would have been considered wheat as little as a century ago.

Today's wheat has been bred to create a crop that generates higher yields and is resistant to disease, drought and heat. In fact, modern wheat has been tinkered with so much that it is unable to grow in the wild without being fertilized and subjected to pest control. It's like a dog that wouldn't be able to survive without a human feeding it special food and taking care of all of its needs.

Wheat has undergone dramatic genetic changes as scientists attempted to produce a strain that would offer high yields. This was achieved via cross-breeding with strains of wheat that contained the desirable characteristics, such as shorter stalks which reach maturity faster. The shorter stalk was also a solution to the problem of high-yields because when wheat was treated with large quantities of nitrogen-rich fertilizer to increase yields, the seed head at the top of the plant grew very large and the original long stalk was unable to support it. Thus, the stalk would buckle under the weight, making harvesting problematic. The shorter stalk was stockier and, therefore, stronger, ensuring the plant could maintain its posture.

The problem is that throughout all these experiments and procedures, no one took the time to determine what impact the resulting crops would have on human and animal health. Scientists were too intent on producing high-yield crops and helping to deal with world hunger that they never stopped to think what they were producing could actually be more harmful than helpful. They simply assumed that they genetically modified crops they were creating were safe for human consumption.

After all, hybridization strategies have been employed for hundreds of years in animals, crops and even people, though in a more primitive form. And the resulting products were all healthy, so why should this be any different? The fact is that these cruder forms of selection didn't change the genetic makeup of the "end-product". Breeding a milk cow with a bull would still create a cow, with the same basic structure, though one that could produce milk. It didn't lead to the birth of a completely different animal, which is pretty much what has happened to wheat.

And things aren't looking up. In the past, scientists would have to cross-breed strains and hope that the result would be what they wanted. Now, though, specific genes can be added or removed deliberately, with wheat being bred to survive in different conditions, including being resistant to cold, drought and more. Basically, scientists can tinker with the genetic code of wheat to create anything they want.

What's worse is that this is big business. Companies can patent their seeds and demand a premium for specific strains. They can even design the crops to be compatible only with certain fertilizers and pesticides, which would boost sales of those particular products. In other words, these companies are making a fortune at the cost of our health, while hiding behind the civilized veneer of "we're helping people" by eliminating famine. Yet, with all these advanced techniques, our greater understanding of genetics and everything we can do, no one has taken a moment to conduct tests on how healthy these genetically modified crops are for humans.

Understanding Wheat

Wheat is commonly referred to as a complex carbohydrate and is touted as being healthy for you. But let's take a look at modern wheat flour and see what's actually going on.

Modern wheat flour made from the Triticum aestivum strain contains 70 percent carbohydrates, with around 10-12 percent each of protein and fiber with the tiny left over percentage being fat, mostly in the shape of polyunsaturated fatty acids and phospholipids.

The starch present in wheat has been named a complex carbohydrate and there isn't a nutritionist who doesn't love it. A complex carbohydrate is one that is made up glucose polymers, in other words repeating chains of simple sugar. Simple carbohydrates like sucrose, on the other hand, are made up of sugar structures with one or two units at most. Most dietitians along with the USDA recommend that we cut down our consumption of simple carbs while increasing the amount of complex carbs we consume.

In wheat, 75 percent of the complex carbohydrate present is comprised of chains of branching glucose units, known as amylopectin, with the remainder being linear chains of glucose units, or amylose. When ingested, these two compounds are digested by an enzyme known as amylase, which is present in saliva as well as the stomach.

Amylopectin is quickly digested by this enzyme and converted into glucose, while amylose is harder to break down, which is why some of it passes through the digestive system whole. So, 75 percent of the complex carbohydrate present in wheat is converted into glucose and quickly absorbed into the bloodstream, causing spikes in blood sugar.

Other foods that contain carbs also present amylopectin but it's not the same as the one present in wheat. Research shows that the structure of this compound differs depending on where it comes from. For example, beans contain amylopectin C, which is the hardest to digest, making its way to the colon intact. The bacteria in the colon then feeds on the starches that haven't been digested and emit nitrogen and hydrogen as well as other gases, which is why beans cause gas. This process, however, ensures that your body can't absorb the sugars present in beans.

Amylopectin B is present in bananas and potatoes and even though it's more digestible than amylopectin C, it still offers some resistance. Amylopectin A is the easiest to digest for our bodies, making it the version of this compound that has a significant impact on blood sugar and it's the one that is present in wheat. This is why wheat has a more significant impact on blood sugar than beans or even French fries.

So, the complex carb that is being touted as the healthiest of them all is easier to convert into glucose causing more significant spikes in blood sugar than practically any other type of carb, be it simple or complex. In fact, the high content of amylopectin A present in wheat makes the latter worse than many simple carbohydrates, including sucrose.

And nothing can make this clearer than the glycemic index, which measures the impact of foods on blood sugar. White bread has a GI of 69, while the GI of whole grain bread is 72. Funnily enough, sucrose registers 59 on the GI scale while a Mars bar has a glycemic index of 68. In other words, eating a Mars bar is apparently better than eating whole grain bread in terms of its impact on your blood sugar. How misleading is the GI scale when you view it this way?

It's also been shown that processing has little to no impact on blood sugar. Wheat is still wheat, regardless of the processes it has been subjected to. Thus, the conclusion is that wheat has the ability to increase blood sugar more than practically any carb, from legumes to chocolate bars. This is important in terms of weight gain because the presence of glucose automatically stimulates the production of insulin, which is a hormone that ensures glucose can enter our cells, transforming it into fat. The more glucose is present in the blood after a meal, the more insulin will be produced and the more fat will be deposited.

This is why it has been shown that a steak does not increase body fat because it doesn't increase blood sugar levels, while a few slices of whole wheat bread increased blood glucose significantly, leading to production of insulin and accumulation of fat, especially in the abdominal area.

Wheat also has another curious behavior in terms of blood glucose spikes. The increase in glucose and insulin caused by amylopectin A is a process that lasts approximately 120 minutes, with a glucose high followed by a drop in glucose. So, you go from being full to feeling hunger pangs within two hours and this process repeats itself throughout the day. This is why you're hungry two hours after eating a wheat cereal breakfast in the morning and why you experience hunger pangs and cravings an hour before lunch. This process is also responsible for fatigue, mental fog and shakiness.

This cycle that triggers high glucose levels followed by increased insulin causes a high level of fat accumulation, which is especially noticeable in the abdominal region, which is why you get "wheat belly". The more fat you have in this area, the higher your resistance to insulin is, which requires even greater insulin amounts to be produced, eventually leading to diabetes.

In men, the more fat they have, the more estrogen is produced by the fat cells and the bigger their breasts grow. The larger your wheat belly, the more susceptible you are to other health issues such as heart disease and cancer.

Thus, according to the Wheat Belly Diet, if you eliminate wheat from your diet, this problem disappears, especially since wheat is also an appetite stimulant because of the cycle generated by amylopectin A. So, if you eliminate wheat from your diet, you will eat fewer calories, which will accelerate your weight loss.

Eliminating wheat from the diet has been proven to induce weight loss as studies on patients with celiac disease have proven. A study conducted at the Mayo Clinic on 215 celiac patients who were obese found that they lost 27.5 pounds within the first six months of eliminating wheat from their diets.

The Wheat Belly Diet: What Is It?

First and foremost, the Wheat Belly Diet is adamant when it comes to eliminating wheat from your diet. Some might find it hard to build a wheat-free life because this grain has made its way into practically every aspect of the modern diet.

For a lot of people, it will require a serious shift in mindset and habits. They'll have to change the ways they shop, cook and eat. Some people think that they'll starve without their cereals, bread, hamburger buns, pasta, cookies, cakes, and other wheat-based products. Some people won't have such a panicked reaction but they'll still feel uncomfortable about it.

Then there are those who will have an actual physical reaction. They will experience withdrawal symptoms that might include cravings, sadness and, in some extreme cases, depression.

So, yes, it might sound tough to eliminate wheat but think of all the benefits. You'll be free of the glucose-insulin-fat cycle that is destroying your health. You'll finally lose the weight that you haven't been able to budge for years and you'll feel more energetic.

Unfortunately, there's no halfway with wheat. You have to get rid of it. Reducing the amount won't cut it. You either go all the way or you don't bother.

Get Ready for Better Health

You have to ignore the nutritionists and USDA claiming that whole grains are healthy for you. These people have spent years telling us that whole grains should be the main part of our diet if we want to feel great, to look amazing, and to be successful and popular. They say that whole grains promote healthy cholesterol levels and regular bowel movements while a deficiency will lead to heart disease, cancer and you will end up malnourished and unhealthy.

Unfortunately, most of what we are being told is backed by agricultural and food companies looking to make a profit. Wheat is one of the cheapest ingredients on the planet thanks to all the genetic modifications and it can be turned into hundreds of different products that sell for a much higher price than the cost of ingredients.

There's nothing better for a company than a product that causes addiction and costs them practically nothing to make and nets them a huge profit. So, of course they are going to lobby to put wheat on the "approved foods list" and market it until you end up thinking that you'll die if you don't eat wheat for a week.

The fact that whole grains are healthy is blatantly untrue and they are in no way a necessity in the human diet. In other words, you can go your entire life without eating wheat and you won't have any problems. In fact, people who don't eat wheat at all tend to have low triglycerides and high levels of HDL or "good" cholesterol, stable blood sugar, stable blood pressure and lots of energy. The typical wheat-free person is also slim, has no abdominal bulge, sleeps well and has normal bowel function.

In other words, there is no such thing as "wheat deficiency syndrome," which is just a term some clever marketers coined to frighten us into buying those wheat products and making sure we eat plenty of it. After all, they have to keep their profits up, don't they? Otherwise, some CEO or VP of marketing won't be able to afford to buy another yacht or mansion this year from the bonuses they made selling us poison.

As long as you replace wheat in your diet with well-considered healthy food choices, a dietary deficiency should not develop after eliminating wheat. It's important to replace those calories with quality foods like vegetables, nuts, meats, eggs, avocados, olives and cheeses. This will lead to improved health, higher energy levels, loss of fat and a better quality of life since you aren't plagued by the numerous ills wheat consumption causes.

However, if you replace wheat with potato chips, candy bars and sodas, then you've eliminated wheat for nothing and you could end up with a deficiency of certain nutrients. Of course, you will continue to gain weight and will more than likely develop other health conditions too, including high cholesterol, high blood pressure and even diabetes.

Thus, the first step is to eliminate wheat and the second step consists of finding quality replacements for the wheat products in your diet. You'll find you naturally eat at least 350 to 400 fewer calories per day, so you won't need as much food to replace all these wheat products you are removing from your diet.

Even if all you do is remove wheat from your diet and eat more of the foods you currently eat, it's still a lot better than continuing to eat wheat. In other words, eat more salad, fruits and vegetables, and include scrambled eggs, baked chicken and tomatoes but drop the wheat.

Wheat Elimination Is Only the First Step

If you want to slim down and achieve excellent health, then simply eliminating wheat isn't going to be enough. You need to make sure you replace the lost calories with quality food. In other words, avoid foods that are processed, treated with herbicides and other chemicals, and genetically modified.

Definitely skip anything that comes in a box and is ready-to-eat. In fact, anything that has a label that reads like a chemical experiment or has an ingredient list with numbers or symbols you don't understand should be avoided, especially those products that require clever marketing campaigns to sell.

Breakfast cereals are sold using cartoon characters and sports figures on clever marketing campaigns to entice more people to eat them, but when's the last time you saw an advertisement for a raw steak?

It's going to take a lot of willpower to cut out all wheat-based foods from your diet, because there's a lot of pressure to eat the foods that are bad for you. All day, you see ads for foods you should avoid and a lot of money is spent on discovering ways to get us to buy more of these unhealthy foods. And all these marketing ploys work, no matter how hard you try to ignore them. But, you have to steel yourself and ignore peer pressure and cut out the processed foods and wheat from your diet. You won't develop any nutritional deficiencies. In fact, you will become much healthier, so don't fall for the hype that's designed to get you to spend your hard-earned cash on food that will destroy your health.

The only real problem with eliminating wheat and processed foods from your diet is convenience. Cooking delicious, nutritious meals from scratch takes a little longer than popping something into the microwave or frying it from a box. However, once you get used to it you might even find you enjoy preparing new recipes. Many people do. And there are plenty of great tasting recipes that take less than 30 minutes to prepare and are very healthy for you. Exploring new recipes, experimenting with spices and herbs and trying new foods is actually fun.

Going Cold Turkey

The Wheat Belly Diet recommends that you quit wheat cold turkey. It's the most effective way to get rid of the problems wheat causes. Additionally, the addictive properties of the glucose-insulin-fat cycle make it difficult for many people to slowly lower their consumption of wheat, in which case an abrupt elimination is preferable.

Simply cutting back can cause more cravings than if you eliminate it completely, which is why it might be easier to deal with withdrawal symptoms. However, if you feel more comfortable, you could *try* cutting back until you've removed wheat completely from your diet.

If you do choose to cut back, though, you have to be honest with yourself. In other words, be realistic on whether you really are cutting back or are simply telling yourself you are. We have a great capacity, as humans, to lie to ourselves so make sure you really are reducing the quantity of wheat you are eating. And, remember, the ultimate goal is to stop eating it altogether.

Look for foods that are labeled "gluten free". These foods don't contain any hidden wheat or cereal fillers to bulk them up and they're designed to be suitable for those people who actually have a physical wheat intolerance. Many of these foods may help you find substitutes when you're cutting the wheat out of your own diet. Just be sure you're still making healthy food choices when you're checking out those labels.

Plan for Success

As previously mentioned, eliminating wheat can be inconvenient. You may have to take your own food to work and will probably require a fork or spoon to eat it because sandwiches and wraps are no longer on the menu. You'll have to buy vegetables, which might mean going to the store, market or greengrocer a few times a week because fresh vegetables don't have an indefinite shelf-life.

And yes, you will have to learn to cook at least a few recipes but you'll probably start enjoying it when you discover what great food you can create that's healthy for you.

Think about what replacement foods you might use to make some of the things you usually enjoy. Rice flour works well in some recipes, as does almond flour, millet, quinoa, arrowroot, gram flour made from chickpeas, and cornstarch or cornmeal. Remember, these are intended as potential substitutes for wheat, but you still need to be sure that you prepare them in recipes that are healthy for you and that won't affect your weight loss efforts. There are plenty of strategies you can employ to succeed.

And before long, you'll find that being alert and full of energy all day long is much more important than eating a doughnut or the five minutes you might save by buying processed food. You'll feel so much better that going back to your old way of eating simply won't be worth it. You will no longer have cravings and won't have to eat constantly to keep your blood sugar elevated so you don't fall into the slump and mental fog the glucose-insulin-fat cycle causes.

You'll be able to go without food for longer and you'll be happy eating less because there's nothing to trigger the need for more calories. You'll naturally eat less and lose weight, which will also boost your self-confidence. It won't be long before you never want to see wheat again.

The Side Effects of Reintroducing Wheat

Once you've avoided wheat for a few months, you might find that starting to eat wheat products again will cause some unpleasant side effects, including aches in your joints, asthma, upset tummy, gas and more. Even if you didn't experience withdrawal symptoms, these problems can still occur.

Generally, people who start eating wheat again experience things such as gas, bloating, cramps and diarrhea, which can last anywhere from six hours to two days. And this can occur from only a few slices of bread.

Taking Your Weight Loss to the Next Level

While removing wheat from your diet will eliminate the biggest problem that might have been stalling your weight loss, even if you were eating only healthy foods, there are other carbs that can cause problems as well. Wheat is the worst carbohydrate but there are others you should cut back on or eliminate completely if you have a lot of weight to lose.

In fact, Dr. Davis recommends an overall reduction of carbohydrates, which will help eliminate the problems caused by a diet with excessive quantities of carbohydrates thanks to all the processed foods people consume.

The following foods should be reduced significantly:

- Cornstarch and cornmeal – this includes wraps, tortillas, corn chips, tacos, corn breads, breakfast cereal and any sauce or gravy in which cornstarch has been used as a thickener;
- Snacks – products like rice cakes, popcorn, potato chips;

- Desserts – if it's got sugar in it, avoid it. So, forego the pies, cakes, ice cream, cookies, and candy bars;
- Rice – a serving of ½ a cup is fine but any more than that, whether it's white, brown or wild rice, will have a nasty effect on your blood sugar;
- Potatoes – white, red or sweet potatoes have the same effect as rice so keep portion sizes small;
- Legumes – kidney beans, lima beans, butter beans, chickpeas and so on. Large servings cause spikes in blood glucose. Once again, keep serving sizes small;
- Foods labeled as gluten-free – the gluten is replaced with cornstarch, rice starch, potato starch or tapioca starch, so be sure you keep serving sizes small and use them only in healthy recipes;
- Fruit juices and soft drinks – You can have small servings of natural fruit juices that don't exceed four ounces but otherwise, you are drinking liquid sugar. You are better off eating the fruit itself as the fiber will help fill you up instead of going right through you. The vitamin C and flavonoid content of fruit juice is not sufficient to justify the intake of so much sugar. Soft drinks should be eliminated completely because of the added sugar, high-fructose corn syrup, colorings and the carbonation;
- Dried fruit;

One thing you need not restrict is fat, as it's been proven to be healthy for you. However, this means **natural** fats. There are certain fatty foods and fats that you need to avoid such as hydrogenated or trans fats, fried oils and cured meats because of their content of sodium nitrate and AGEs.

What to Eat

The Wheat Belly Diet recommends including the following foods to your diet:

Vegetables
These are the best foods on the planet as they are rich in nutrients, vitamins and minerals, and should be the main component of your diet. There are lots of vegetables you can try, so be sure you experiment with different recipes and styles. You're bound to find some that you like and with a little creativity in the kitchen, you can turn any vegetable into an amazingly tasty dish. And don't limit your vegetable intake to dinner. Work on ways to include more vegetables into other meals as well.

Fruit
The Wheat Belly Diet recommends a limited intake of fruit because most fruits are too rich in sugar, mainly due to genetic manipulation. So, have a small serving of fresh fruit like berries, which have a lower sugar content than any other fruit and the highest nutrient content. Fruit like bananas, pineapple and mangos should be enjoyed once in a while, but not every day.

Raw nuts
These are filling and have a high content of monounsaturated oils, protein and fiber, which are all healthy for you. They can help reduce blood pressure and LDL cholesterol. They may also have a beneficial effect in slowing down aging. However, all the nuts you consume must be raw, not roasted in oil, honey roasted, beer nuts or any other type of processed nut.

Oils
You don't have to limit your intake of oils. In fact, you can use healthy oils such as extra-virgin olive oil, coconut oil, avocado oil and coconut butter generously. However, you should avoid polyunsaturated oils such as sunflower, safflower, corn and vegetable oils.

Meat, Poultry and Eggs
Eat plenty of chicken, turkey, lean meat and eggs, including sirloin and pork. It's been proven that saturated fat is not the problem when it comes to cholesterol and heart disease, but saturated fat in combination with carbohydrates. In fact, the major problem was discovered to be carbs. Try to buy organic meat and avoid frying it. Also, stay away from cured meats. You can eat as many eggs as you want as there is no restriction. Your body will tell you what it wants because your appetite signals will start behaving naturally after you eliminate wheat.

Dairy Products
You can enjoy full-fat cheeses as well. There are a wide range of cheeses you can eat but stick to full-fat because low-fat ones are often bulked up with starches and their taste improved with sugar, which will negate all your efforts. So, eat Cheddar or Swiss or try something that might be new to you like Edam, Roquefort, Stilton, Brie, and Camembert and so on. Cheese can be a great snack or the main component of a meal. It can also be used to flavor dishes, giving them a completely new dimension.

Other types of dairy, such as cottage cheese, yogurt, milk and butter should be limited to one or two servings per day. This is because they have a high content of dairy proteins, which tend to increase the production of insulin.

Is The Wheat Belly Diet Right For Me?

The Wheat Belly Diet, essentially, recommends eating healthy whole foods, and that can only be beneficial, regardless of whom you are. Eliminating wheat will have no harmful effects on you and you can only benefit from it.

There are no health conditions that will be negatively impacted by the elimination of this grain and even vegetarians will do well to eliminate it. In fact, many vegetarians or vegans don't lose weight because they replace animal proteins with wheat products and processed foods, which actually cause them to gain weight.

The only way to really tell if this diet will work for you is to try eliminating wheat for at least a month or two. If you only give it a week, you may experience withdrawal symptoms that won't let you accurately assess how you feel on this eating plan.

In any case, you should focus on eating whole foods and eliminating processed foods from your diet, whether or not you choose to cut wheat out. However, the author of this diet makes a good case for the elimination of wheat and you can only benefit from it. You'll likely experience an increase in energy levels, if nothing else, so it's definitely worth giving this diet a go.

Wheat Belly Diet vs. Healthy Eating and Exercise

The Wheat Belly Diet recommends healthy eating and healthy food choices. However, it doesn't mention exercise whatsoever, which is remiss of the author. The diet itself doesn't focus only on weight loss but on promoting good health.

To achieve good health, some physical activity in your daily routine is essential.

So, while you will lose weight just by following the diet, you still incorporate an exercise plan to achieve the best results.

Exercise will help tone your muscles, which will boost your metabolism and increase the number of calories your burn at rest. This means you will lose weight faster. The extra muscle will also help you avoid the thin "flabby" look many people sport because they don't exercise at all.

Additionally, regular exercise will improve your mood and your energy levels. At first you might think that you don't have enough time to exercise but if you cut out half an hour of television per day, you'll have enough time to exercise.

Or you can even exercise in front of the TV and even if it might seem hard at first, your energy levels will soon skyrocket and the endorphins released during exercise will have you looking forward to it.

Think about looking into some easy, quick and effective incidental exercises. These are things you do throughout your day that aren't actual planned workouts. They're short and simple, but they can be seriously effective for toning your body and helping to lose weight.

Tips to Succeed with the WHEAT Belly Diet

Here are a few tips to help you succeed with the Wheat Belly Diet.

Plan

The key to succeeding with the Wheat Belly Diet is to plan. You won't be able to eat sandwiches or wraps and you'll have to cook for yourself. So, plan in advance. There are plenty of options when it comes to food you can take to work. You can cook in bulk and freeze portions so you can have food for the week without having to spend time every day cooking.

Drink Water

Water is essential to the functioning of the body and it will help flush out toxins as well as keeping you hydrated. Hunger pangs can sometimes be confused for thirst, so getting enough water will help you eat less, without realizing it or making any effort to do so.

Don't Shop on an Empty Stomach

Eat before you go grocery shopping. When you're hungry you are more likely to give in and buy foods that you should be avoiding. But if you've eaten beforehand and go shopping on a full stomach, it will be easier for you to make rational decisions.

Forget About Wheat

You have to forget about wheat and processed products based on wheat. If you think of this diet as something you'll try for two weeks and then go back to eating bread and cereal, there's no way you will succeed. You need to think of it as a lifestyle change.

You Are Human

You have to allow yourself to make mistakes. IN other words, if you've slipped up, don't throw in the towel and go all out. It will be weeks before you start your diet again and you'll never lose the weight. Instead, accept that you are human and will make mistakes and just move on. Jump right back on the bandwagon because eating healthily 90 percent of the time is better than trying to be 100 percent but never doing it.

Conclusion

The Wheat Belly Diet presents a good case for the elimination of wheat. However, the author does emphasize that eliminating wheat alone will not help you achieve the weight loss results you want.

Instead, this diet is focused around eating healthy foods. There's sufficient variety to keep you from getting bored and there are no restrictions on calories though you will likely be eating less because protein and fat tend to make you feel full for longer.

So, there's no harm in eliminating wheat from your diet. You only have to gain from getting rid of this much-maligned carbohydrate. The increase in energy levels and the lack of the afternoon slump should be incentive enough for you to adopt a wheat-free diet, let alone the weight loss you should experience.

If you can also find ways to get some incidental activity into your daily routine, you should find that your weight loss results are staggering.

Good luck!

BONUS CONTENT PREVIEW OF THE 15 MINUTE GUIDE TO INCIDENTAL EXERCISE

INTRODUCTION

If you really hate to exercise, you'll be very pleased to know that you can improve your fitness levels, burn fat, improve your health, tone up your body, get rid of cellulite and lose weight just with some simple incidental activity spread out through your regular daily routine.

The key to really making incidental activity work for you is to look for opportunities. Don't see moving your body as a chore. Instead, think of every opportunity as a bonus. It's just another way you get to look and feel great without going to the gym.

Start a Biggest Movers contest with yourself. To get you to think differently, researchers say we have to see a reward. So why don't you think of three things you've been wanting and give yourself a little challenge before you get it. It can be anything: a pedicure, a new fragrance, a magazine, music CD or a book. But before you buy it give yourself a milestone to hit.

If I get 3 incidental activities done today, I'll give myself_____. Just fill in the blank with your hearts desired item.

If I find 5 incidental activities today, I'll get my pedicure Friday the 14th of May at _____.
A secret to getting yourself to take action on this is to stack the odds in your favor. How? By calling, scheduling it in and living as if you've already done it.

If I complete 21 days of incidental activities, I can add $50 more dollars to my Financial Freedom Funds.

I think you get the picture. Once you own this process and make it yours you'll find yourself thinking up ways to get more rewards. This is exactly the motivation we all need and respond to since ancient days. Now, take a look at the incidental activities that work like magic.

Walking

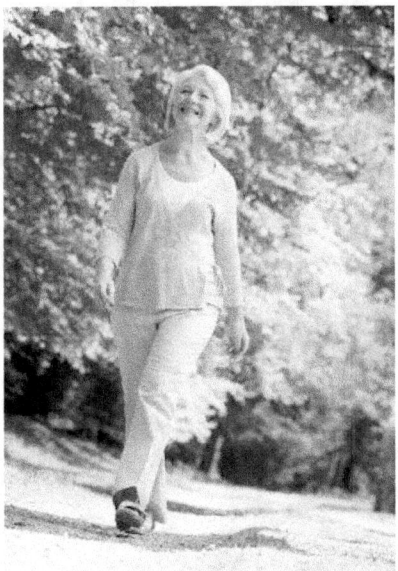

Let's be honest: not many people have the time or the inclination to walk around the neighborhood block for 30 minutes after a long day at work. This type of suggestion just doesn't work with most busy, modern families.

Instead you can use incidental activity to get your daily walking done. After all, six individual 5 minute walking sessions still adds up to 30 minutes so you're getting the same results overall.

The next time you're in the car searching for a car parking spot, don't try to circle around and look for a parking spot as close to the doors as you can find. Instead, find a park spot that is a bit further away and walk that extra minute or two to your destination. You'll find that it's always quicker and easier to find a park spot this way and you're getting those extra steps in without much effort.

Don't drop the kids off right in front of the school. Park a short distance away and walk with them. If your kids don't want you walking all the way to the school, you might want to stop a little distance away to be sure they get there before you walk back to the car.

If a friend calls you on the phone, don't drop onto the sofa to enjoy a good chat. Instead, why not pace around the room while you talk?

Always remember to stand with your back straight whenever you walk. Hold your head high and suck in your abdominal muscles as you walk. This helps to tone your stomach with every step you take and improves your posture at the same time.

Every day you should be able to find a couple of small opportunities to get even a few extra steps into your daily routine. These all accumulate to a daily total that helps you get closer to your goals.

Laughing

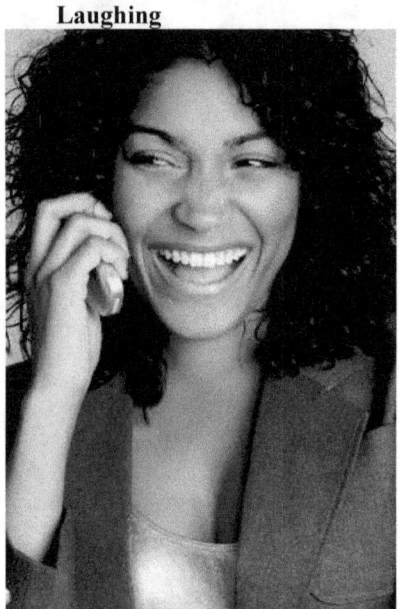

One of the easiest and most fun incidental exercises of all is laughing. Did you know that when you laugh your body is expending energy? A good old-fashioned belly laugh causes muscle contractions within your abdomen, so you're naturally using more energy to make that happen. You're also helping to tone those abdominal muscles when you really get into a good belly laugh.

Research has shown that laughing 100 times burns the same amount of energy as spending 15 minutes on an exercise bike. I don't know about you, but I'd much rather laugh my way through a silly comedy movie or hang out with friends who make me laugh than ride an exercise bike for 15 minutes!

Aside from this, when you laugh your body releases endorphins. These are your body's natural 'feel-good' chemicals. Runners get a 'runners high' because of the endorphin rush. You don't have to run, just laugh more, so you should find that you reduce stress levels naturally and you're in a better mood as a result.

Watching TV

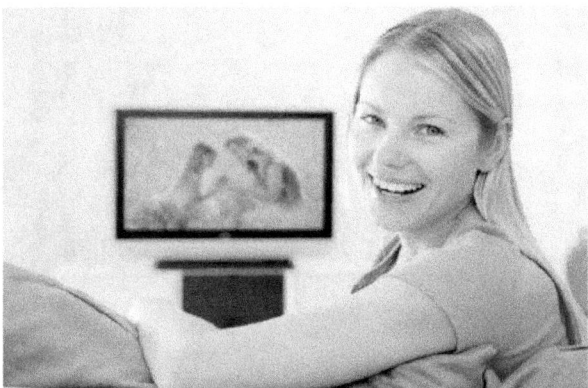

Who would have believed you can boost your fitness and tone your body while you sit on the sofa watching TV? Yet you can. The whole point of incidental exercise is to get your body moving. If you're moving, you're expending energy.

Fidget while you sit. Wobble your legs while you wait for a green light or let your foot swing back and forth while you watch your favorite show.

If you want to get a bit of body toning work done while you sit, use every commercial break as an opportunity to flatten your stomach and work on your abdominal muscles. When the ad break begins, make an effort to sit up straight in your seat. Pull your stomach muscles in tight, as though you're trying to draw them back towards your spine and hold that position for a few seconds.

This helps to strengthen your stomach and back muscles. Over time, you should notice it becomes much easier to do. You'll be improving your posture at the same time too.

Another option is to tone your butt during the break. Wait for the commercial break to start, then sit upright in your seat. Then clench your butt cheeks together tightly and hold that position for a few seconds before letting go. Repeat this activity until the ads end and your show returns. You'll be tightening and toning your butt while you sit. Terrific!

That is it for the free bonus content. If you'd like to read more about the 15 Minute Guide to Incidental Exercise, just order the book from the place where you purchased the first one.

Best wishes,
Patricia